THE ART OF
LIVING FOODS

ANURA DESAI

Desai Health and Wellness
2440 16th St, NW
Washington, DC 20009
www.desaihealthandwellness.com

This cookbook is dedicated to my loving mother Bhadra, and father Ashok Desai, to my supportive twin brother Urnav, and older brother Mihir Desai, and to my aunt and confidant Rashmi Desai.

TABLE OF CONTENTS

ACKNOWLEDGEMENTS

Recipes for this cookbook were made possible by the generosity of the following cooks. Each cook draws upon their unique talent to create nourishing foods filled with the best ingredient of all, love:

- Anne Elixhauser. Columbia, MD.
- Bhadra Desai. Washington, DC
- Kasia Fraser. Boone, NC
- Kailash Sharma. Quebec, Canada
- Sage Houston. Uvalde, TX
- Shubhu Joshi. Vancouver, Canada
- Viswanathan Umapathy and Rathi Ramamurth. San Francisco, CA

Designed by: Kazaan Viveiros

Food styling by: Kasia Fraser

Editing by: Mihir Desai, Michaela Krna and Kazaan Viveiros

Photography by: Nathan Jackson, Kasia Fraser and Ruben Gamarra

Food photo shoot location: Art of Living City Center, Boone, NC

In deep gratitude to Rajshree Patel, my inspiration, and to Philip & Kasia Fraser, my home

In my mid twenties, I found myself in an unhappy and unsatisfying job, feeling weighed down by challenging health issues, by my self-judgments, and by exhaustion in my body and mind. I couldn't sleep, was constantly worried, and I had also developed a rare vision condition—not at all the life I had envisioned for myself. But this was all transformed in such a simple, yet powerful way.

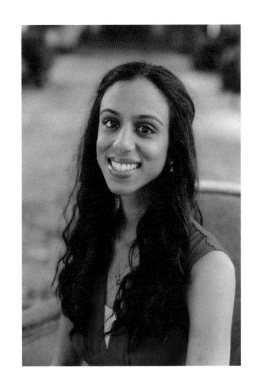

I began spending time in the kitchen of the Art of Living Center in Washington, DC. The Art of Living Foundation is a non-profit that was founded by Sri Sri Ravi Shankar. With only a slight appreciation for food and no experience with cooking, I began making meals to support the various courses in meditation, yoga and well-being held there. With the other volunteers at the Center, I made delicious and flavorful meals for hundreds of people per day.

I learned to savor and appreciate food in a whole new way. I felt an immediate connection with the bright colors, tastes and textures of the fruits, vegetables, herbs, grains and lentils that were being used in simple ways to create wonderful dishes. I realized that simple, natural foods, when combined, provide pleasure and are a powerful source of energy and healing.

I also developed a deep respect for the other volunteers, who are living examples of service, and felt so grateful to support the course participants who, like me, were confronting their own struggles and opening themselves to new possibilities. It was the first time I forgot to worry about myself, or whether I was good enough. Through it all, I learned to simplify, and became part of something much bigger than myself.

Shortly after, the Institute for Integrative Nutrition provided a platform to channel this revived energy. The training gave me a deep knowledge of food and nutrition and prepared me to become a health and wellness coach. I now inspire people to eat and live healthier, so they can regain energy back in their lives. It all started with creating the simple, delicious recipes that fill this book. With gratitude for the grace and presence of Sri Sri in my life and deep appreciation for this experience, I proudly share this cookbook with you.

ABOUT THIS BOOK

I'm so happy to share with you a variety of simple and easy-to-make recipes that I think are delicious and full of the natural energies that give us health, balance and well-being. These meals emphasize whole, living foods such as fruits, vegetables, herbs, whole grains, and nuts/seeds. Meals that incorporate these foods can create lightness, vitality and stamina in our bodies, and calmness, alertness and steadiness in our minds. Living foods give us energy in abundance, allow our bodies to function properly and maintain a healthy weight. Most of all, they are incredibly full of flavor! Each recipe in this book is accompanied by a quote by Sri Sri Ravi Shankar.[1] I hope that you'll enjoy the cookbook and its recipes as much as I do.

FOUR SOURCES OF ENERGY

Just as our experience with food can enhance our energy and help us bring our mind to the present, we also obtain energy from three other sources: Sleep, Breath, and Meditation.

Food is a vital source of energy. When we eat too much, we can feel slow, lethargic and inert. While if we eat too little, our energy levels drop immediately. The quality of food also has an influence. Foods that are old, frozen, processed or contain chemicals offer little energy. Whereas, foods that are organic, fresh, and whole increase our energy. Being aware of adequate quantities, appropriate meal times, and the quality of foods are all essential for providing energy.

Sleep also has a direct physical sensation of energy in our body. When we do not get enough sleep or get too much sleep, our energy is low. Getting adequate sleep enables balance between activity and rest. Turning off electronic gadgets an hour before bed, going to sleep before midnight, and sleeping for six to eight hours ensures quality rest.

Breath is one of the more subtle and constant sources of energy. The act of living itself is directly related to our breath, and yet it often goes unnoticed. The breath connects our mind and body. Each rhythm of breath has a corresponding emotion. When angry or fearful, our rhythm of breath is mostly shallow, and when calm and relaxed, our rhythm of breath is long and deep. Practicing breathing exercises allows us to bring calmness and a sense of relaxation back to the mind. Toxins in the body are released mainly through the breath. When we use our lung capacity to its fullest by way of proper breathing exercises, it allows the body to restore itself.

Meditation uplifts our energy and distributes it outwards. When our mind is calm and steady, it allows us to perceive situations as they are, helps us be alert and decisive, and most of all, it gives us a bright and positive feeling of ourselves and our environment. This type of energy from meditation is the most subtle, deep, and long-lasting. When energy remains contained or suppressed, it can lead to blockages in the physical body and disturbances in the mental body. Low energy and/or stress shows up in different places in the physical body, whether in the back, neck, head, shoulders, muscles, joints or gut. Low or suppressed energy in the body shows up as an overactive, agitated, or depressed mind. Meditation allows energy to move up and out.

THE ENERGETICS OF FOOD

When we eat, we do not measure the quality of the food based on calories or nutrition, but rather based on the experience it gives us. All food contains energy, and that energy creates the living experience in our body and mind. It can either increase energy in the body and mind, or decrease it. Foods that decrease energy include sugars, caffeine and alcohol. These foods give the experience of jitteriness, shakiness and instability in the body, and anxiety, tenseness, and agitation in the mind. Conversely, foods that increase energy include fruits, vegetables, herbs, whole grains, and nuts/seeds. These foods give the experience of lightness, vitality and stamina in the body, and calmness, alertness and steadiness in the mind.

We can approach food with this understanding to influence the experience we have in our body and mind. If we are feeling tense or anxious, eating foods that are grounding such as sweet potatoes, parsnips, and carrots, which are all root vegetables, rooted to the ground, can help. Similarly, if we experience lethargy or inertia, eating foods that are light, such as leafy greens, raw vegetables, and fruits that have grown up and out toward the sun, can help. Choosing a variety of foods provides balance to both body and mind.

Each season in the year provides food aligned with the nature of our environment and our bodies. In the wintertime, when it is cold, dry and airy, nature provides heavier and heartier foods like root vegetables, which warm and nourish the body and ground the mind. In the summertime, when it is hot, humid and stagnant, nature provides lighter and hydrating foods that bring coolness and flexibility to the body, and creativity to the mind. Eating foods aligned with the rhythm of nature helps promote natural balance within our bodies and minds.

The way food is prepared also influences our energy. Foods that were prepared in a microwave, by way of factory farming, or were genetically modified, all contribute to the degradation of cellular structure, which comprises the food's energy. Whereas, eating from your own garden, locally, organically, and cooked over a stove, all help to maintain the freshness, pureness and nutrition of food.

Being aware of the energy that food provides helps us to make better choices when growing or buying food, when preparing food, and knowing when and how to eat it. The energy of food is the best measure of nutrition for our body and mind.

LIVING FOODS

As with most things in life, our knowledge of food comes from wisdom already found deep within us. Our modern, fast-paced lifestyles have impeded our ability to tap in and be guided by this inner knowledge. Reverting back to a simpler approach can unravel the complexities of food—and of life.

The path to simplicity is obtained by balancing our food choices. Choosing whole, living foods rather than processed ones, such as packaged foods full of unrecognizable ingredients, is essential. Choosing from a variety of these living foods throughout the day can ensure that we get the full spectrum of nutrition.

Vegetables offer minerals, vitamins, and fiber to the body. Energetically, they bring about either lightness or a feeling of groundedness. Dark, leafy greens, such as kale, spinach, Swiss chard, dandelion, collard greens, mustard greens, beet greens, bok choy, and watercress are just a few of the varieties that provide lightness to the mind and body. Greens that are eaten raw include romaine lettuce, mesclun, wild greens, arugula, endive, and chicory. Vegetables that are grounding include root vegetables such as beets, carrots, turnips, parsnips, sweet potatoes, and yams. Many of these grounding vegetables are sweet, and can replace sugary, processed foods to satisfy sweet cravings.

Fruits are vital to cleansing our body of accumulated toxins. Rich in antioxidants and fiber, fruits give nourishment to cells and help maintain good functioning of organs. Fruits are energizing, refreshing and can also help to stave off sweet cravings. Choose from a colorful assortment of fruits, such as strawberries, raspberries, blueberries, gooseberries, kiwi, papaya, apple, mango, oranges, banana, cherries, peaches, nectarines, and melons.

Herbs and Spices offer culinary diversity with their strong flavor and enhancement of taste. They also have deep medicinal properties that serve as powerful agents for healing. Herbs and spices help us feel connected to the Earth and nature. Just a little bit can go a long way in any healthy dish. Common herbs include basil, coriander, mint, parsley, oregano, rosemary, thyme, sage, chives, dill and asafoetida. Spices include turmeric, cumin, mustard seeds, black pepper, cloves, ginger, cinnamon, cardamom and nutmeg.

Whole grains are a fixture in any cuisine in every culture. They are a great source of vitamins, minerals, iron, fiber, and enzymes. Since they digest slowly in the system, whole grains provide steady and long-lasting energy. Examples of whole grains are brown rice, quinoa, oats and oatmeal, buckwheat, barley, amaranth, couscous, corn meal, millet, wheat berries, and bulgur.

Protein is essential to maintain cell structure and function in our bodies and makes up much of our nervous system. Proteins provide us with strength, stability, and alertness. Good sources of protein include nuts, seeds, grains, beans, and leafy greens.

In our diets, the more we eat from these living food sources, the less we require in overall food intake. In our lives, the more we engage in activities of service and truth, the less we require in life. Keep food and life simple.

MINDFUL EATING

Eating with awareness is an integral part of our body's ability to absorb the vital energy in food. If we are distracted, agitated or hurried, it diminishes the pleasure that food gives us and the nutrition it provides for the body. The practice of mindful eating brings our attention to the present, drawing upon all our senses for a full experience. There is no right or wrong way to eat, but rather what is present for the individual, mentally, emotionally and physically. Judgment, self-criticism and/or guilt around food do not serve us, and take away from the opportunity for nourishment. Cultivating mindfulness or awareness facilitates our natural ability to know what is best for our own body.

Paying attention to each of our senses while eating allows for presence of mind:
Sight: Look at the food on your plate as if it is your first time eating. Without labeling it, notice the colors, shapes and sizes. Imagine the vital energy within the food.

Smell: Gently bring the food close to your nostrils. Without designating its scent, allow yourself to take in its aroma and temperature.

Physiological reaction: Even before the process of eating begins, notice the reaction in your mouth and stomach at the sight and smell of food.

Touch: Allow yourself to experience the touch of food, how it feels as you hold it. Pay attention to its texture.

Taste: Place the food in your mouth. Feel the sensation on your tongue, and how it naturally moves to one side of your mouth. Bite into your food and focus your attention on what is happening. What is the experience? Notice the flavors—is it sweet, sour, salty, bitter, pungent or astringent?

Texture: As the flavors begin to change and diminish, you will naturally become aware of its texture and consistency. See if you can continue chewing even past the urge to swallow.

Swallow: Move beyond the sensation to swallow. Keep chewing until the body signals the impulse to swallow. Focus your attention on the food as it moves past the mouth, through the throat, and into your stomach. Notice the feeling of food in your body.

Breath: Take pause for a moment to settle into the sensation of food in your body. With the same gentle awareness as you give to seeing, smelling, touching, and tasting your food, pay attention to your breath.

Silence: Without distraction or conversation, allow yourself to take in the experience in silence. Let your body and mind cherish the nourishment your food gives you.

PRAYER TO FOOD

We receive food with gratitude as blessings from the Divine or Nature. We consume it with awareness of the connectedness to the whole of the Universe.

Brahmarpanam Brahma Haviha

Brahmagnau Brahmana hutam

Brahmaiva Tena Gantavyam

Brahma Karma Samadhina

om shaanti shaanti shaanti hi.

We offer this food to the Divine,

This food itself being Divine,

The fire that consumes it being Divinity

and Divine is the act of consuming,
Originating from Divine, this
food and the devoted act of offering
with honor and equanimity,
Culminates in Divinity itself.

In the company of others:

Om sahanaa vavatu Sahanau bhunaktu
Saha veeryam karavaa vahai
Tejasvi naa vadhee tamastu maa vidvishaa vahai
Om Shaanti Shaanti Shaantihi

May we protect each other,
May we nourish each other,
May we work together with great energy,
May our study be enlightening and fruitful,
May we never hate each other,
Om Peace, Peace, Peace.

References:

"What Sri Sri Said Today." Wisdom from Sri Sri Ravi Shankar. The Art of Living Foundation. 28 May, 2012.

15 April, 2012 <http://www.artofliving.org/what-sri-sri-said-today>.

Verma, Krishan. Sri Sri Yoga: A Basic Practice Manual. India: Art of Living (Diamond Books), 2010.

Rosenthal, Joshua. Integrative Nutrition. New York: Integrative Nutrition Publishing, 2007.

BEVERAGES

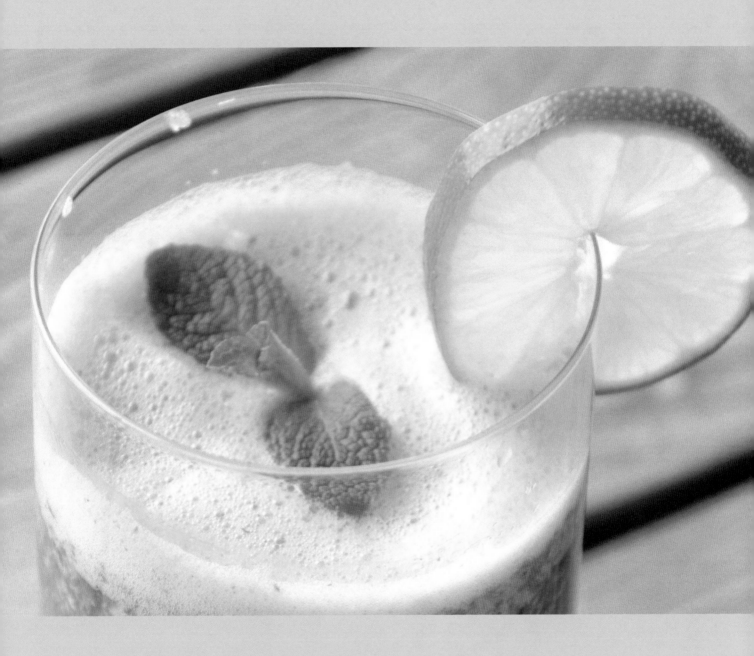

CUCUMBER LIME MINT WATER

1 cucumber, diced

juice of ½ lime

4-6 mint leaves, plus extra leaves for garnish

1 cup water

a pinch of salt (optional)

maple syrup or agave to taste

Blend all ingredients together.
Serve cool.

Serves 1-2

 The food of spirituality is love, joy, compassion and beauty.

LEMON GINGER TEA

¼ teaspoon fresh ginger, grated

a pinch of black pepper

a pinch of tulsi powder (Indian basil - optional)

1 cup water

juice of ¼ lemon

1 teaspoon honey (or maple syrup)

Boil ginger, black pepper, tulsi powder in water. Add lemon juice and honey. Serve hot.

Serves 1-2

 Your body has got enough capability to adjust itself.

WINTER PUNCH

1 cup cranberries
1 cinnamon stick
2 whole cloves
4 cups water
½ cup orange juice, freshly squeezed
½ cup maple syrup
2 lemons, thinly sliced
pinch of nutmeg

Cook cranberries, cinnamon stick, and cloves in water until the cranberry skins pop. Remove cinnamon stick and cloves. Add freshly squeezed orange juice and maple syrup, and boil for 2 minutes. Sprinkle with nutmeg and garnish with lemon slices. Serve hot.

Serves 3-4

 When we eat our food everyday, we must remember with gratitude the farmer who has worked for it.

GREEN SMOOTHIE

2 bananas, roughly cubed
2 cups dark leafy greens, loose
1 heaping teaspoon almond butter
1 heaping teaspoon coconut oil
almond milk

Put bananas, greens, almond butter and coconut oil in blender. Pour almond milk over all ingredients to cover. Blend on medium-high until all ingredients combine to smooth, green color.

Serves 1-2

 One has to listen to their own body. What they feel is good for them.

BREAKFAST

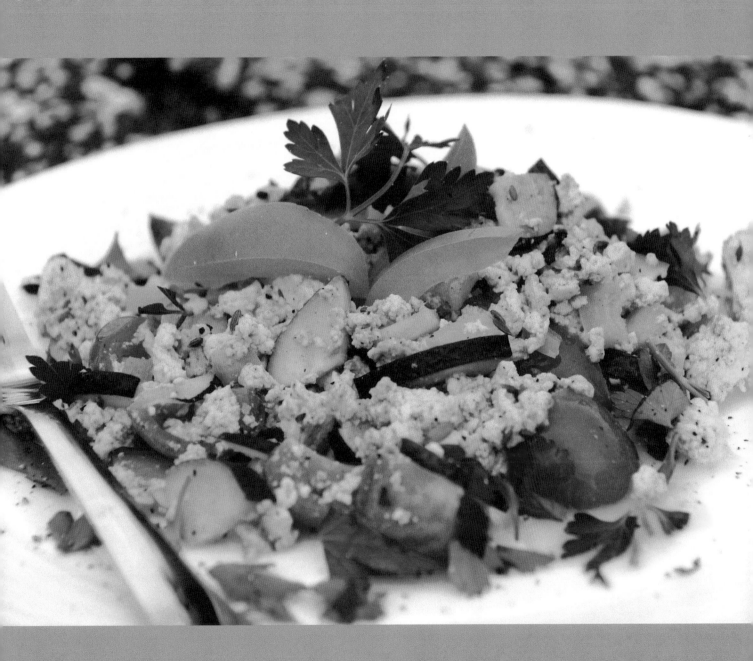

OATMEAL

1 cup oats

2 cups water

½ apple, chopped

¼ cup walnuts, chopped

¼ cup raisins

salt to taste

choice of milk

maple syrup or agave to taste

Boil water. Add oats, apples, raisins, walnuts, and salt to taste. Cook until soft. Serve with your choice of milk. Add sweetener to taste.

Serves 3-4

 There is a proverb which says,
"The one who knows about food does not get diseases."

UPMA

2 tablespoons ghee or olive oil

½ teaspoon mustard seeds

½ cup chana dal

4 curry leaves

½ cup split urad dal

½ inch ginger, grated

½ teaspoon cumin seeds

½ cup green beans, chopped

½ cup peas

2 medium carrots, chopped

3 cups water

½ bunch spinach leaves

1½ cups cream of wheat (semolina) or wheat rava

salt to taste

a handful of cashews

a dash of lemon juice

chopped coriander leaves for garnish

In a pan, heat olive oil on medium. Add mustard seeds and let them pop. Add chana dal, curry leaves, urad dal, ginger and cumin seeds. Cook until all ingredients are golden brown. Add green beans, peas and carrots. Sauté for 5 minutes. Add water. Once boiling, add spinach and cream of wheat, and stir continuously. Add salt. Reduce heat and cook uncovered for 10 minutes. Add extra water, if too dry. Add cashews. Garnish with lemon juice and coriander. Serve hot.

*Can be made with steel-cut oats, as well.

Serves 3-4

 Food is important when you are hungry and unimportant when you are full. When something is inevitable you don't categorize it as important or unimportant. It is beyond choice. "Everything is important" is karma yoga. "Nothing is important" is deep meditation.

TOFU SCRAMBLED

16 ounces (1 block) firm tofu

1 tablespoon olive oil

¼ teaspoon cumin seeds

salt to taste

¼ teaspoon turmeric

½ cup red bell pepper, chopped

½ cup zucchini, chopped

black pepper to taste

Press tofu to remove excess water and crumble into small pieces. In a pan, heat olive oil on medium, add cumin seeds and cook until golden brown. Add tofu, salt and turmeric. Sauté for 5 minutes. Add red pepper, zucchini, and black pepper. Cook for 5 more minutes or until mixture is thoroughly heated.

Serves 3-4

Moderate food and moderate activity makes you realize that you are connected to the universal spirit. Then you don't feel you are just a human being, but realize you are much bigger. The body is a small thread, the mind is much bigger. Our mind is occupying the whole universe. The mind is much bigger and the consciousness is so vast.

POHA (FLATTENED RICE)

2 cups thick poha

2 tablespoons lemon juice, freshly squeezed

2 tablespoons olive oil

½ teaspoon mustard seeds

½ teaspoon sesame seeds

¼ teaspoon turmeric powder

¼ teaspoon asafoetida

1 green chili, finely chopped (optional)

2 tablespoons cashews, finely chopped

1 sprig curry leaves

2 tablespoons cranberries or raisins (optional)

1 large potato, diced

¼ cup coriander, chopped

salt to taste

black pepper to taste

Place poha in colander and gently rinse for 2 minutes. Set aside to drain. Sprinkle salt and lemon juice over poha and gently mix with a fork.

In a pan, heat olive oil on medium. Add mustard seeds and let them pop. Add sesame seeds, turmeric powder, asafoetida, green chili, cashews, curry leaves and cranberries. Sauté for 1 minute.

Add diced potato to the above mix and cook until tender. Fluff up poha and add to the pan. Mix well. Sprinkle with a little water if poha has dried out too much. Garnish with chopped coriander and serve hot.

Serves 3-4

 That is what it is.
Whatever is on my plate today is the best food for today.

SALADS

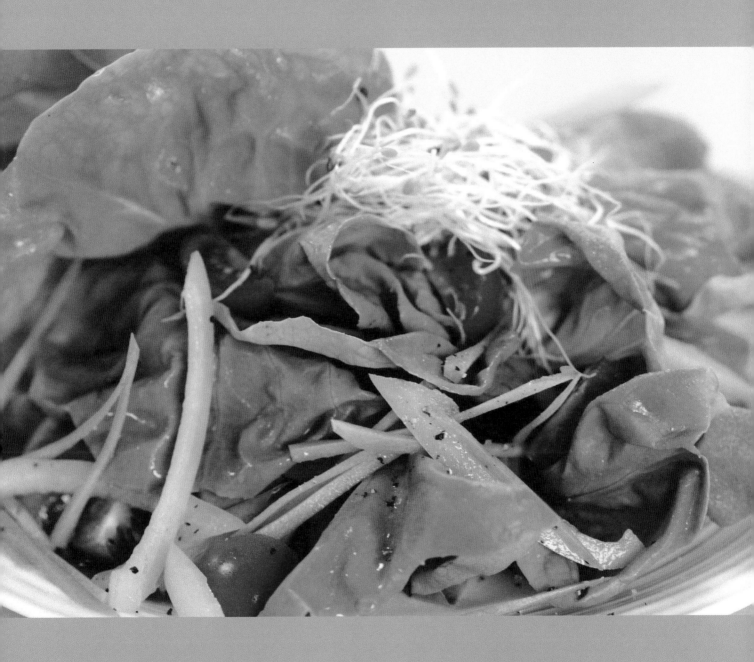

BEET AND GOAT CHEESE SALAD

4 large beets

6 ounces (1 bag) arugula salad

1 ounce goat cheese

¼ cup fresh basil

¼ cup orange juice

3 tablespoons honey

¼ cup ginger, grated

½ cup olive oil

salt to taste

black pepper to taste

chopped fresh basil for garnish

Steam beets until soft, let cool, then remove skin and cut into one-inch cubes. In a salad bowl, mix arugula, crumbled goat cheese and beets. In a separate bowl, mix all ingredients for dressing. Pour over salad mix to coat. Garnish with fresh basil and serve immediately.

Serves 3-4

 Yoga, Pranayaman, Meditation, Ayurveda and eating food which is grown organically, we must resolve to incorporate these into our life.

ITALIAN SALAD WITH GRAPE POPPY SEED DRESSING

6 ounces (1 bag) Italian salad mix

½ cup sweet grapes

¼ cup olive oil

1 tablespoon lime juice

1 teaspoon poppy seeds

1 teaspoon fresh rosemary

½ cup water

salt to taste

black pepper to taste

Mash grapes (with skin on), and heat on stove for a few minutes. Remove from heat and strain through a cheesecloth to make fresh grape juice. Mix juice together with remaining dressing ingredients in a blender. Pour on salad mix and toss to coat. Serve fresh.

Serves 3-4

 Food, food, food. Change your food habits!

ITALIAN SALAD WITH ORANGE DRESSING

¼ cup orange juice, freshly squeezed

½ teaspoon orange zest

maple syrup to taste

3 tablespoons olive oil

½ cup yellow bell pepper, chopped

½ cup cucumber, chopped

1 carrot, shredded or cubed

6 ounces (1 bag) Italian mixed greens

raisins for garnish

Mix juice, zest, syrup and olive oil in blender. Wash and chop bell pepper, cucumber and carrot and add to Italian mixed greens. Pour dressing over salad and toss to coat. Sprinkle raisins on top. Serve immediately.

Serves 3-4

 People who are too finicky about food, their immune system keeps on getting weaker and weaker. When something challenging is given to the immune system, it gets a chance to work....

SPINACH QUINOA SALAD

2 cups quinoa, cooked

½ cup almonds, sliced and roasted

1½ cups spinach leaves, finely chopped

¼ cup fresh cherries or raisins

½ cup cucumber, chopped

½ cup chickpeas, cooked

½ cup celery, chopped

1 avocado, diced

2 tablespoons yogurt

¼ cup olive oil

a dash of fresh lemon juice

¼ inch ginger, grated

salt to taste

black pepper to taste

Mix quinoa, almonds, spinach, cherries, cucumber, chickpeas, celery and avocado in large serving bowl. Whisk together yogurt, olive oil, lemon juice, ginger and salt in small bowl. Pour over salad and toss to coat. Season with black pepper to taste. Serve fresh.

Serves 3-4

... So now and then, once in a while, the immune system should be challenged. Then the self defense will come up from within.

MIXED SALAD WITH AGAVE MUSTARD DRESSING

6 ounces (1 mixed bag) salad greens

½ cup celery, chopped

½ cup red cabbage, chopped

½ cup cucumber, chopped

2 tablespoons agave

2 tablespoons mustard

3 tablespoons olive oil

salt to taste

black pepper to taste

Mix greens, celery, cabbage and cucumber.

Mix or blend all dressing ingredients, pour over salad and toss to coat. Serve fresh.

Serves 3-4

 ...Being finicky gives rise to frustration and anger. Your system should be flexible and adjustable. And that can happen when you resolve mentally that the type of food you are going to eat won't affect your system too adversely...

ARUGULA AND STRAWBERRY SALAD

6 ounces (1 bag) arugula salad

½ cup strawberries

½ cup walnuts

1 ounce goat cheese

2 tablespoons strawberry preserves

¼ cup balsamic vinegar

2 tablespoons olive oil

1 tablespoon water

salt to taste

Mix arugula, strawberries, walnuts and goat cheese. Mix or blend all dressing ingredients, pour over salad and toss to coat. Serve fresh.

Serves 3-4

...That doesn't mean eat unhealthy food. But that means not to be too finicky about food and quality of food. Chose a middle path.

ITALIAN SALAD MIX WITH BASIL LIME DRESSING

6 ounces (1 bag) Italian mixed greens

2 cups cucumber, chopped

1 cup celery, chopped

1 cup tomatoes, chopped

½ cup olive oil

½ cup lime juice

4 tablespoons lime zest

10 basil leaves, chopped

1 tablespoon agave

salt to taste

Mix salad greens with cucumber, celery and tomatoes. Mix together olive oil, lime juice, lime zest, basil and salt. Pour over salad.

Serves 3-4

 After having food, if you sleep on your left side, the right nostril will work, which will aid in digestion.

INDIAN SALAD WITH POMEGRANATE

1 cucumber, chopped

1 tomato, chopped

1 cup cabbage, chopped

1 beet, chopped

1 carrot, chopped

¼ cup yellow bell pepper, chopped

¼ cup orange bell pepper, chopped

2 tablespoons pomegranate seeds

salt to taste

black pepper to taste

½ teaspoon cumin powder

juice of ¼ lemon, freshly squeezed

¼ cup coriander leaves

Put all the vegetables in a mixing bowl. Add pomegranate seeds, salt, pepper, cumin powder, lemon juice and coriander leaves. Mix well and serve fresh.

Serves 3-4

 You know, the impact of food doesn't stay for too long. Minimum, it stays for 24 hours and maximum, for 3 days. That is it, and then it goes away.

SOUPS

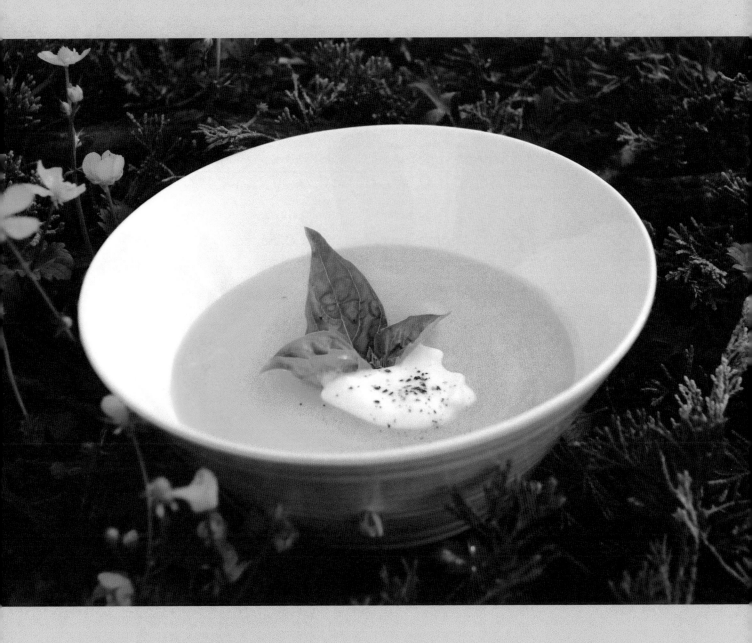

PUMPKIN FENNEL BULB AND SWEET POTATO SOUP

½ pumpkin, chopped

½ cup fennel bulb root, chopped

2 sweet potatoes, chopped

2 cups water

salt to taste

black pepper to taste

2 tablespoons olive oil

1 teaspoon nutmeg

1 sprig sage

Cook pumpkin, fennel and potatoes in water with salt and pepper. Tip: Do not put too much water, just enough to cover the vegetables slightly. Once soft, blend with hand blender, and add olive oil and nutmeg. Garnish with sage and serve hot.

Serves 3-4

 Eating the wrong food or vata aggravating food, eating at odd times, not exercising, and overworking can all cause a physical restlessness. The remedy for this is exercise, moderation in work habits, and going on a vegetable or juice diet for one or two days.

1 squash, chopped

2 red bell peppers, chopped

8 asparagus spears, chopped

1½ cups water

2 tablespoons olive oil

salt to taste

black pepper to taste

chopped coriander leaves for garnish

Cook squash, red peppers and asparagus in water with olive oil, salt and pepper. Tip: Do not put too much water, just enough to cover the vegetables slightly. Once soft, blend the soup halfway. Gently mix. Simmer for 5 to 8 minutes. Garnish with coriander and serve hot.

Serves 3-4

 If you take good precaution with food and you're eating habits are good, you don't get diabetes, or blood pressure or heart problems...

BUTTERNUT SQUASH SOUP

1 large butternut squash, cubed

1½ cups water

½ cup milk (can be almond or soy)

2 tablespoons olive oil or ghee

salt to taste

black pepper to taste

fresh basil for garnish

Cook butternut squash in water with salt. Tip: Do not put too much water, just enough to cover the vegetables slightly. Cook until soft, blend with hand blender, add olive oil (or ghee), milk and black pepper. Simmer for 5 to 8 minutes. Garnish with fresh basil.

Serves 3-4

 Prana (life force) is linked to energy and linked to the space you are in. It is also linked to food, to the breath, to vibrations and energy in the body.

ZUCCHINI SOUP

4 zucchini, chopped

1½ cups water

salt to taste

2 tablespoons olive oil or ghee

½ cup milk (can be almond or soy)

black pepper to taste

fresh dill for garnish

Cook zucchini with water and salt. Tip: Do not put too much water, just enough to cover the vegetables slightly. Once soft, blend with hand blender. Add olive oil (or ghee), milk and black pepper. Simmer for 5 to 8 minutes. Garnish with fresh dill and serve hot.

Serves 3-4

 Though the river is vast, a little sip quenches your thirst. Though Earth has so much food, just a little bite satisfies your hunger. All that you need is teeny, tiny bits. Accept a teeny tiny bit of everything in life, which will bring you fulfillment.

BARSZCZ (BEET SOUP)

3 beets, chopped

3 potatoes, chopped

2 carrots, chopped

1 celery stalk, chopped

1 parsley root, chopped

2 tablespoons olive oil

salt to taste

½ inch ginger, grated

3 beet leaves, chopped

black pepper to taste

3 tablespoons fresh lemon juice

1 cup yogurt (optional)

2 cups water

fresh dill for garnish

Cook all vegetables in water with olive oil, salt and ginger. Once soft, blend together with hand mixer. Add beet leaves, pepper and lemon juice. Simmer for 5 to 8 minutes. Garnish with fresh dill. Serve with yogurt (optional).

Serves 3-4

 Balance in activity, balance in food and balance in your rest, your sleep, will bring equilibrium within you.

THAI COCONUT SOUP

3 yams, chopped

2 carrots, chopped

2 tomatoes, chopped

3 lemongrass stalks

2 cups water

1 can coconut milk

2 tablespoons fresh ginger, chopped

½ bunch basil, finely chopped

salt to taste

black pepper to taste

Cook yams, carrots, and tomatoes in water. Tip: Do not put too much water, just enough to cover the vegetables slightly. Blend with hand blender until smooth. Cut lemon grass and boil in 2 cups water. Add coconut milk and ginger and let boil for 15 minutes. Add blended vegetables to coconut milk mixture to bring it to a soup consistency. Continue boiling for 5 minutes. Add salt, pepper, and finely chopped basil. Serve hot.

Serves 3-4

 As you keep growing older, keep practicing yoga, take proper food, proper rest, and adopt a proper attitude in life.

CARROT SOUP

6 large carrots, chopped

1 celery stalk, chopped

1 tomato, chopped

½ inch ginger, grated

1 teaspoon cumin powder

salt to taste

black pepper to taste

½ cup cashews (optional)

2 cups water

½ cup orange juice

chopped coriander leaves for garnish

Soak cashews and grind into a paste. Cook carrots, celery and tomato in water with ginger, cumin powder, salt and pepper. Tip: Do not put too much water, just enough to cover the vegetables slightly. Once soft, blend together with cashews and orange juice. Garnish with coriander and serve hot.

Serves 3-4

 Sudarshan Kriya, meditation, some yoga and proper food will take care of [of an overactive mind].

MIXED VEGETABLE SOUP

1 cup mung dal	Wash and soak mung dal in water with a pinch of salt for one hour, drain.
3 cups water	
3 carrots, chopped	
½ cup green beans, chopped	Cook mung dal in 3 cups water. Once soft, use hand blender to mix thoroughly. It should not be too thick. Add vegetables and cook until soft. Add tofu. Add fresh basil, olive oil, salt and pepper. Simmer for 5 to 8 minutes. Serve hot.
1 sweet potato, chopped	
2 zucchini, chopped	
½ block tofu (optional)	
2 tablespoons olive oil	
salt to taste	
black pepper to taste	
fresh basil for garnish	Serves 3-4

 The food habits that we have in our country are not good for memory power because we eat so much starch...and so little vegetables. So, change your diet. Have more intake of proteins, vegetables and fruits, and some ayurvedic supplements like brahmi, etc. This, along with your pranayama and yoga, will improve memory.

TOMATO BLACK OLIVE & CHICKPEA STEW

½ cup chickpeas

2 cups water

2 tablespoons olive oil

1 cup whole peeled tomatoes, chopped

½ cup black olives, pitted

1 teaspoon oregano

½ inch ginger

salt to taste

black pepper to taste

fresh lemon juice to taste

Soak chickpeas in water with a pinch of salt for one hour, drain. Cook chickpeas with 2 cups water and use lid to cover the pot halfway. Allow to simmer for one hour, until soft. In a pot, heat olive oil on medium. Once hot, add tomatoes, chickpeas, olives, oregano, ginger, salt and pepper. Add water. Cook for 15 minutes. Set aside, covered, until ready to serve. Add lemon juice to give it a slightly tangy taste.

Serves 3-4

 At the body level, desires are influenced by the chemical responses in your body due to your food, water, environment, your age and the company you keep.

BUTTERNUT AND PUMPKIN SOUP

1 butternut squash, peeled and cubed

½ pumpkin, peeled and cubed

2 tablespoons olive oil or ghee

¼ teaspoon mustard seeds

½ teaspoon cumin seeds

1 teaspoon turmeric

½ inch ginger, grated

1 teaspoon nutmeg

3 tablespoons lime juice (or apple juice)

½ cup rice milk

salt to taste

parsley for garnish

Cook butternut squash and pumpkin in water with salt. Tip: Do not put too much water, just enough to cover the vegetables slightly. Once soft, blend together with hand mixer. In a pan, heat olive oil on medium, and add mustard seeds. Once mustard seeds pop, add cumin seeds, turmeric, ginger and nutmeg until brown. Mix spices with soup. Add juice and milk. Simmer for 10 minutes. Garnish with parsley and serve hot.

Serves 3-4

 Telling people to be vegetarian, they don't feel like listening to that. But it happens naturally when you become subtle in your mind and go deep in your heart, you turn vegetarian naturally. The more refinement in the system, the system wants light food [that] is easily digestible.

1 cup red lentils

½ cup barley

3 cups water

2 tablespoons olive oil or ghee

½ teaspoon mustard seeds

1 teaspoon cumin seeds

1 teaspoon turmeric

½ inch ginger, grated

2 carrots, chopped

juice of 1 lemon

salt to taste

black pepper to taste

½ cup baby spinach leaves

chopped coriander leves for garnish

Soak lentils in water with a pinch of salt for one hour, drain. Cook lentils and barley in 3 cups water, until soft. Then blend with hand blender until smooth. In a pot, heat olive oil on medium. Add mustard seeds and cook until they pop. Add cumin seeds, turmeric and ginger. Sauté for 1 minute. Add carrots and sauté until slightly cooked. Add lentil and barley mixture. Allow mixture to boil. Season with salt and black pepper, adding enough water to achieve a soup consistency. Add spinach and lemon juice. Garnish with coriander and serve hot.

Serves 3-4

 Junk food can also block your mind. Have confidence that everything will be okay - this is number one, then prayerfulness ... and then proper food and rest, pranayam and yoga—all this will help.

VEGAN SPLIT PEA SOUP

1 cup dried split peas
½ cup barley
3 cups water
2 carrots, chopped
2 celery stalks, chopped
1 sweet potato, chopped
2 tablespoons olive oil
2 bay leaves
1½ teaspoons thyme
salt to taste
black pepper to taste
fresh parsley for garnish

Wash and soak split peas in water for one hour. Cook peas and barley with 3 cups water and salt for 25 minutes, or until soft. Boil vegetables in small amount of water with olive oil, bay leaves, salt and black pepper. Once soft, remove bay leaves, add peas and barley. Mix together. Add thyme. Garnish with parsley and serve hot.

Serves 3-4

 Too much food makes you feel dull. Meditation doesn't happen then. Moderation, don't fast also, just the right amount of food.

WHOLE MUNG SOUP

1 cup whole green mung	Soak mung beans in water with a pinch of
3 cups water	salt for one hour. Drain, then cook mung
2 tablespoons olive oil or ghee	in 3 cups water for 25-30 minutes, or until
1 teaspoon cumin seeds	soft. In a pan, heat olive oil on medium.
1 teaspoon cumin powder	Add cumin seeds, roast for half a minute.
3 tablespoons fresh lemon juice	Add cumin seed mixture to mung beans.
salt to taste	Add cumin powder, lemon juice, and salt to
chopped coriander leaves for garnish	taste. Garnish with coriander and serve hot.

Serves 3-4

 You know, what is the latest finding of non–vegetarian food? One kg of meat is equivalent to the meals of 400 people. If only 10 percent of the world population become vegetarians, the problem of global warming will be reduced. On this count, we have to save the planet.

YELLOW MUNG SOUP WITH KALE

1 cup yellow mung

3 cups water

2 tablespoons olive oil or ghee

½ inch ginger, grated

1 teaspoon cumin seeds

2 teaspoons garam masala

1 teaspoon cumin powder

1 teaspoon turmeric

4 tablespoons coconut flakes, dried

3 tablespoons fresh lemon juice

2 cups kale leaves, chopped

salt to taste

chopped coriander leaves for garnish

Soak mung beans in water with a pinch of salt for one hour. Drain, then cook mung in 3 cups water for 25-30 minutes, or until soft. Once soft, more water can be added for desired consistency. In a thick bottom pan, heat ghee with ginger and add cumin seeds. Cook until brown and add sautéed mixture to soup. Add garam masala, cumin powder, turmeric, coconut flakes and lemon juice. Cook for 5 minutes and add kale leaves. Garnish with coriander. Serve hot with rice.

Serves 3-4

 God has given us the sense to care for others and the planet, also! You have eaten enough, so consume a little less, so that others who have nothing to eat can have a little at least, so that more and more people get something to eat.

MOROCCAN SPICED VEGETABLE STEW

2 red potatoes, peeled and chopped

1 medium butternut squash, chopped

2 carrots, chopped

½ cup tomatoes, diced

½ cup garbanzo beans, cooked

2 tablespoons olive oil

2 teaspoons cumin powder

salt to taste

1 cup water

½ teaspoon red pepper flakes

¼ cup raisins

chopped coriander leaves for garnish

In a pan, sauté chopped vegetables and garbanzo beans with olive oil, cumin powder and salt. Add one cup water to soften. Use lid to cover the pot halfway. Once soft, add red pepper flakes and raisins. Garnish with coriander. Serve hot with rice or bread.

Serves 3-4

We have to care for the whole planet. We have to make the entire planet organic. When it comes to making food, growing food, you cannot say, "OK, I'll grow organic food only in this part and other parts can be polluted with chemicals," because the air will carry!

VEGETABLE SOUP

1 russet potato, chopped
6-8 almonds, blanched
1 cup broccoli florets
½ cup coconut milk
¼ cup leeks, chopped
¼ cup parsley, chopped
1 sprig sage
a pinch of nutmeg
salt to taste
black pepper to taste

Cook all vegetables together with almonds, salt and pepper, until soft. Tip: Do not put too much water, just enough to cover the vegetables slightly. Blend with hand mixer until smooth, add coconut milk. Simmer for 5-10 minutes. Season with parsley, sage and nutmeg. Serve hot.

Serves 3-4

 I think every individual, every human being on the planet, will have to take the responsibility of not polluting the planet, of continuing sustainable development by planting more trees, preserving our lakes, preserving water. It is so important!

VEGETABLES

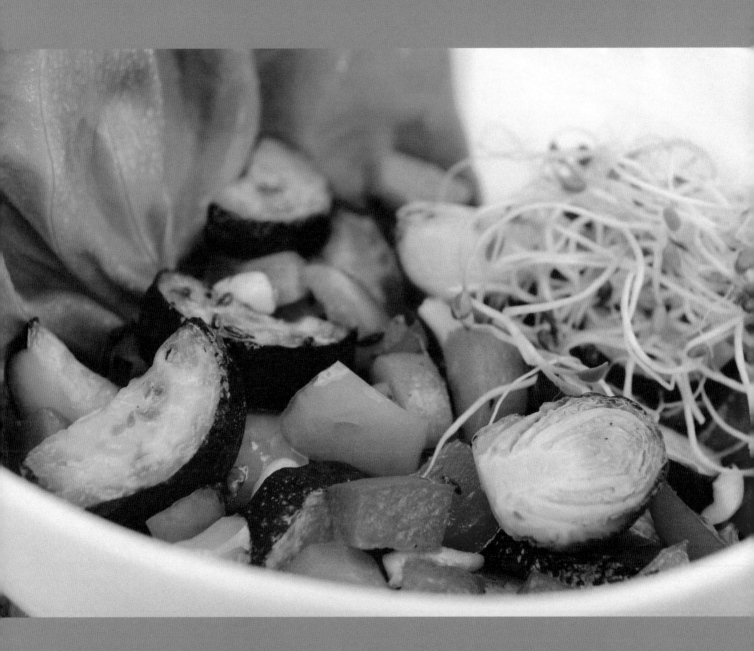

ROASTED ROOT VEGETABLES

2 cups rutabaga, chopped into 2 inch pieces

2 cups parsnips, chopped into 2 inch pieces

2 cups carrots, chopped into 2 inch pieces

¼ cup olive oil

2 tablespoons fresh basil, chopped

salt to taste

black pepper to taste

¼ cup parsley for garnish

Pre-heat oven to 425 degrees. Boil cut vegetables for 5 minutes, then drain water. Pour olive oil into baking dish and place in oven for 5 minutes.

Mix vegetables with basil, salt, and pepper. Pour vegetables into hot olive oil. Roast for 30 minutes, turning every 10 minutes. Garnish with parsley and serve hot.

Serves 3-4

 Our food influences our mind.

GARBANZO-STUFFED SQUASH

2 acorn squash, cut in half
2 granny smith apples, finely chopped
1 can garbanzo beans
1 teaspoon Herbs de Provence
salt to taste

Bake halved acorn squash for 30 minutes in pre-heated oven at 350 degrees. While squash is baking, sauté apples, beans, herbs and salt. Cover and cook until apples are soft. Stuff squash with mixture and serve hot.

Serves 3-4

 Modern science confirms that food can have a direct bearing on our emotions.

ZUCCHINI BABA GHANOUSH

3 zucchini, chopped
½ cup tahini sauce (sesame paste)
juice of 1 lemon, freshly squeezed
salt to taste
black pepper to taste

Bake zucchini in pre-heated oven for 30 minutes at 375 degrees. Once soft, blend with tahini, lemon juice, salt and pepper. Serve warm or cold.

Serves 3-4

 We offer prayers before eating. The food that we eat absorbs the vibrations. Respecting food means respecting farmers. We should always keep in mind that the one who is producing food should always be happy, because that is the origin of the thought cycle. This is our beautiful tradition.

VEGETABLE CASHEW CURRY

2 tablespoons olive oil

16 ounces (1 block) firm tofu

½ inch ginger, grated

1 teaspoon cumin seeds

2 bell peppers

½ cup green peas

½ cup cashews

2 tomatoes

3 curry leaves

1 teaspoon turmeric

salt to taste

black pepper to taste

1 teaspoon cumin powder

¼ cup water

½ cup olive oil

½ can coconut milk

chopped coriander leaves for garnish

In a pan, heat olive oil on medium. Sauté tofu, ginger, salt and cumin seeds until slightly brown. Add bell peppers and green peas, and sprinkle with some water, if necessary. Blend cashews, tomatoes, curry leaves, turmeric, salt, pepper, cumin powder, water and olive oil in a blender. Add paste to tofu. Add coconut milk and simmer for 8-10 minutes. Garnish with fresh coriander.

Serves 3-4

 Food makes us experience the chaitanya (the consciousness). That is why it is called *Brahman*.

SWEET POTATOES AND PECANS

3 large sweet potatoes, peeled and cubed

¼ teaspoon turmeric

salt to taste

1 teaspoon cumin powder

2 tablespoons olive oil or ghee

½ cup pecans, roasted

½ cup raisins

In a pan, heat olive oil on medium. Sauté sweet potatoes with turmeric, salt and cumin powder until soft. Add roasted pecans and raisins. Serve immediately.

Serves 3-4

 The type and amount of food that we consume has a direct impact on the state of our physical body, and consequently, our mind.

ROASTED BRUSSELS SPROUTS

2½ cups brussels sprouts
3 tablespoons olive oil
salt to taste
black pepper to taste
5 tablespoons white miso
3 tablespoons maple syrup

Trim sprouts and mix with olive oil, salt and pepper. Spread onto baking sheet and bake for 20 minutes in pre-heated oven at 375 degrees, until sprouts are slightly brown. Mix together white miso and maple syrup. Remove brussels sprouts from oven. Pour white miso and maple syrup mixture on sprouts. Place sprouts back in oven for another 10 to 15 minutes. Serve hot.

Serves 3-4

 Observe what you eat. Fresh fruits and vegetables have more prana (life force), while frozen and canned foods have very little prana.

SAUTÉED GREEN VEGETABLES WITH PESTO

2 tablespoons olive oil
1 cup green beans, chopped
2 cups broccoli, chopped
1 cup zucchini, chopped
½ cup fresh basil
½ cup pine nuts (or cashews)
½ cup olive oil
salt to taste

In a pan, heat 2 tablespoons olive oil on medium. Sauté green beans, broccoli and zucchini with salt. Cover to cook thoroughly. Sprinkle with some water to aid cooking process. For pesto, blend basil, pine nuts, olive oil and salt in a blender. When vegetables are tender, toss with pesto from blender. Serve hot.

Serves 3-4

 Different types of food that you take influence you for some days.

GREEN BEANS WITH COCONUT

2 tablespoons olive oil

½ teaspoon cumin seeds

¼ teaspoon asafoetida

¼ teaspoon turmeric powder

1 teaspoon fresh ginger, grated

¼ cup powdered or grated fresh coconut

5 to 6 curry leaves

1 teaspoon coriander powder

¼ teaspoon cumin powder

salt to taste

3 cups green beans

½ cup water

fresh lemon juice to taste

chopped coriander leaves for garnish

In a pan, heat olive oil on medium and add cumin seeds. Once the cumin seeds pop, add asafoetida, turmeric powder, ginger, coconut, curry leaves, coriander powder, cumin powder and salt.

Add green beans to the pan with the spices and water. Cook for 10 minutes, until the beans are soft. Add lemon juice and mix. Garnish with coriander leaves and serve hot.

Serves 3-4

 Food is connected with God. In the Upanishads, it is said 'Food is God.' When you consider food as God, you will not over eat. You don't simply stuff food, but you eat food with so much honour.

LECHO

½ cup chickpeas
2 tablespoons olive oil
1 sweet potato, cubed
½ inch ginger, grated
1½ teaspoons cumin seeds
¼ teaspoon turmeric
salt to taste
2 carrots, chopped
1 yellow squash, chopped
1 red bell pepper, chopped
1 yellow bell pepper, chopped
parsley for garnish

Wash and soak chickpeas overnight, at least 5-6 hours, until softened. Cook chickpeas with water and salt until soft, drain. In a pan, heat olive oil on medium and sauté sweet potatoes, ginger, cumin seeds, turmeric and salt. Add some water to aid the cooking process. Add carrots, yellow squash, red and yellow peppers and cooked chickpeas. Cook until soft, adding more water, as needed. Garnish with fresh parsley. Serve hot.

Serves 3-4

 You know people in poor areas, slums especially—I am talking about India—they are so much stronger. Their immune system is very strong and their body is like steel. You will be surprised...

INDIAN SQUASH (LOKHI) AND ASIAN SWEET POTATOES

1 small Indian squash
1 medium Asian sweet potato
2 tablespoons olive oil
¼ teaspoon mustard seeds
¼ teaspoon cumin seeds
¼ teaspoon asafoetida powder
½ teaspoon garam masala (optional)
½ teaspoon turmeric powder
½ teaspoon fresh ginger, grated
¼ teaspoon cumin powder
1 teaspoon coriander powder
1 sprig curry leaves
salt to taste
½ cup water
chopped coriander leaves for garnish

Wash and peel squash and sweet potato and cut into ½ inch cubes. In a pan, heat olive oil on medium and add mustard seeds. After the mustard seeds pop, add cumin seeds, asafoetida and garam masala. Add turmeric, ginger, cumin powder, coriander powder, curry leaves and salt.

Mix squash and sweet potato cubes and add to the pan with the cooked spices. Add water, cover and cook, until vegetables are tender. Let the mixture simmer for about 10 minutes. Garnish with chopped coriander and serve hot.

Serves 3-4

... People who are in urban areas, their system is a little weak. You catch cold, you get a cough when you go to some polluted areas. But these people who live in slums, they are so robust. Their immune system is so strong, because it is active. It is very strange, but true.

VEGETABLE STIR FRY WITH TOFU

1 extra firm tofu, cubed

2 tablespoons olive oil

½ inch ginger, grated

salt to taste

1 red bell pepper, diced

2 carrots, sliced

1 zucchini, sliced

1 head broccoli, chopped

¼ teaspoon turmeric

juice of 1 lemon

1 teaspoon maple syrup

chopped coriander leaves for garnish

In a pan, heat olive oil on medium. Sauté tofu with ginger and salt. Add vegetables and turmeric. Once soft, add maple syrup and lemon juice. Garnish with coriander and serve hot.

Serves 3-4

 If you are always eating super healthy food, sometimes your body loses its capacity to adjust and your immune system becomes a little weak. So, you should make your body flexible. Sometimes you can eat not too healthy food... it doesn't have to be organic all the time...Your body has the ability to adjust to every situation.

VEGETABLE WRAP

1½ cups walnuts or almonds, chopped

1 cup dill, chopped

juice of ½ lemon

1 teaspoon salt

a dash of Bragg's liquid amino acid

½ cup olive oil

5 tablespoons water

4 whole wheat wraps

2 cups bell peppers, cut into long, thin slices

1 cup carrots, cut into long, thin slices

1 cup celery, cut into long, thin slices

Blend together nuts, dill, lemon juice, salt, Bragg's, olive oil and water to a smooth paste. Spread paste on half of each wrap. Place raw vegetables on top of paste. Roll wrap from vegetable side and serve fresh.

Serves 3-4

 Follow the middle path. Take healthy food most of the time, but sometimes be used to other food, as well.

GRAINS

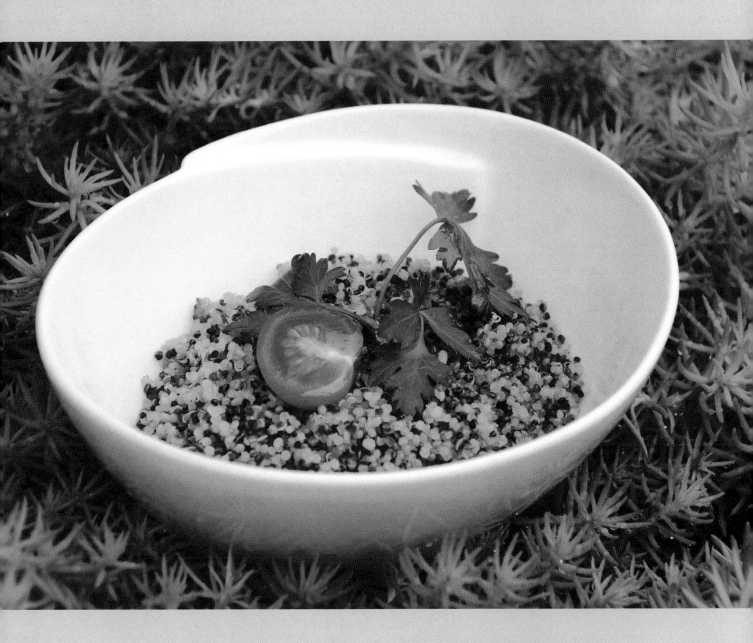

ISRAELI COUSCOUS WITH VEGETABLES

2½ cups cooked Israeli (pearl) couscous

2 teaspoons olive oil

½ cup currants or raisins

½ cup dried apricots

½ teaspoon salt

42 ounces vegetable broth (or water)

3 cinnamon sticks

¼ cup coriander leaves

In a pan, heat olive oil on medium. Sauté couscous for 2-3 minutes. Stir in currants, apricots, salt, broth (or water), and cinnamon sticks. Bring to a boil. Cover, reduce heat, and simmer for 15 minutes. Let couscous stand for 5 minutes. Discard cinnamon and stir in coriander. Serve hot.

Serves 3-4

Too much knowledge all at once cannot be digested. Knowledge should be given in small doses, like in a five course dinner: first the appetizer, then the soup, then the main meal and in the end, dessert. This way we can digest the food.

½ cup masoor dal

½ cup yellow dal

½ cup quinoa

½ cup barley

1 tablespoon rye flakes

½ cup millet

2 tablespoons olive oil

¼ teaspoon mustard seeds

¼ teaspoon cumin seeds

¼ teaspoon fenugreek seeds

½ teaspoon crushed red pepper (optional)

¼ teaspoon turmeric

1 teaspoon coriander

½ teaspoon paprika

6 cloves

½ cup tomatoes

½ cup carrots

½ cup zucchini

a handful of green beans

¼ cup cabbage

a handful of asparagus

salt to taste

Cover masoor dal, yellow dal, quinoa, barley, rye flakes and millet with water and cook, adding more water as necessary to maintain consistency. In a separate pan, heat olive oil on medium and add mustard seeds, cumin seeds, fenugreek seeds, crushed red pepper, turmeric, coriander, paprika and cloves. Add vegetables to the pan and sauté with spices for a few minutes, then pour into the cooked legumes and grains. Add salt to taste. Stir and simmer for a few more minutes. Adjust seasoning before serving.

Serves 3-4

 There is a proverb in India, 'A spoonful of ghee (clarified butter) on rice purifies the rice.' You know why? This is because if you eat rice just like that, it digests very fast and becomes sugar very quickly. Many people who eat rice like that, they become diabetics.

KALE AND CHARD QUINOA

1 cup quinoa

1½ cups water

4 leaves kale, finely chopped

4 leaves chard, finely chopped

2 teaspoons Indian curry powder

½ cup lemon juice

salt to taste

chopped coriander leaves for garnish

In a pot, boil quinoa in water with a pinch of salt. In a separate pan, heat olive oil on medium and sauté kale and chard. Add Indian curry powder and salt. Add cooked quinoa and lemon juice. Garnish with finely chopped coriander and serve hot.

Serves 3-4

 A cardiologist told me, anytime you [eat] cereal you should have a little bit of fat with it. A spoon of ghee on top ... slows down the digestion. It becomes complex carbohydrates and helps to balance the sugar level in the body, and that helps a healthy heart function.

LEMON MINT BASMATI RICE

1 cup basmati rice

2 cups water

1 teaspoon cumin powder

salt to taste

2 tablespoons olive oil

½ teaspoon cumin seeds

¼ teaspoon turmeric powder

juice of 1½ lemons, freshly squeezed

½ cup mint leaves, finely chopped

Cook rice with 2 cups water. Once cooked, transfer to a bowl and add cumin powder and salt to taste. In a separate pan, heat olive oil on medium and add turmeric and cumin seeds. Pour over rice. Add lemon juice and mix well with a fork. Garnish with mint leaves. Serve hot.

Serves 3-4

 Eating the right types and amounts of food promotes all-around well-being and can increase energy levels [and] help us manage stress more effectively.

PASTA

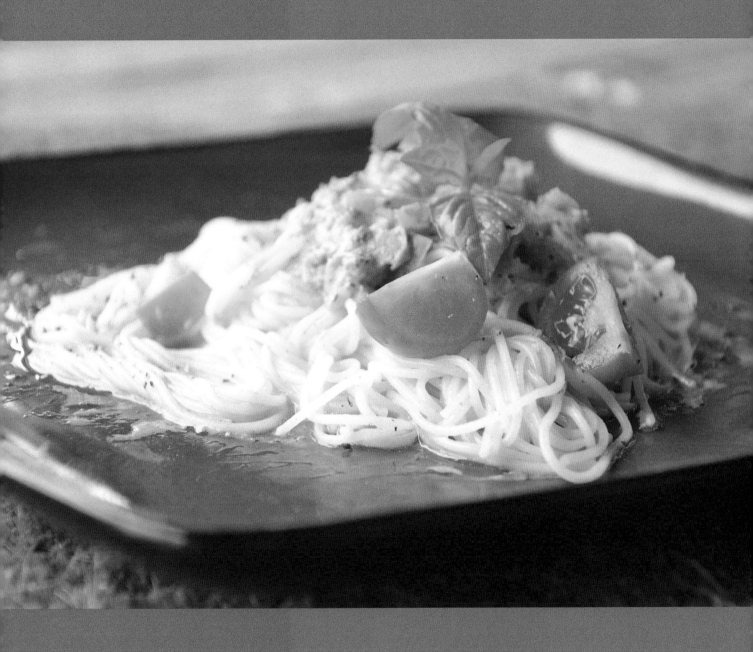

PASTA WITH CREAMY VEGETABLE SAUCE

8 ounces whole wheat pasta
1 cup carrots, chopped
1 cup zucchini, chopped
2 ripe tomatoes, chopped
1 cup leafy greens
½ cup blanched almonds
½ cup olive oil
2 teaspoons basil
1 teaspoon oregano
salt to taste
black pepper to taste

Cook pasta according to box directions. Boil carrots and zucchini in a pot with tomatoes, and cover with water, approximately 2 inches above the vegetables. When cooked, add almonds, olive oil, basil, oregano, salt and black pepper. Blend together all ingredients to a sauce consistency. Pour over whole wheat pasta. Add leafy greens and serve hot.

Serves 3-4

 Music is food for the emotions; Knowledge is food for the intellect; Meditation is food for the soul.

PASTA WITH SPAGHETTI SQUASH SAUCE

8 ounces whole wheat pasta

1 spaghetti squash, cut in half and deseeded

1 cup tomatoes, diced

1 cup leafy greens

½ cup olive oil

½ bunch fresh basil

salt to taste

black pepper to taste

Cook pasta according to box directions. Bake spaghetti squash in pre-heated oven at 350 degrees. When soft, scoop out the squash pulp. Cook tomatoes and leafy greens in a pan and add the squash pulp. Mash ingredients together with a fork or hand blender. Add olive oil, basil, salt and black pepper. Pour over whole wheat pasta. Serve hot.

Serves 3-4

 Different kinds of vegetables should be grown. One should have knowledge of food.

PASTA WITH ITALIAN TOMATO SAUCE

8 ounces whole wheat pasta
1 extra firm tofu, cubed
1½ cup carrots, chopped
1 head broccoli, chopped
2 zucchini, chopped
1½ cup ripe tomatoes, diced
salt to taste
black pepper to taste
½ cup Italian herbs

Cook pasta according to box directions. In a pan, heat olive oil on medium. Sauté tofu, carrots, broccoli, zucchini and tomatoes. Add salt and black pepper. Add Italian herbs, and blend all ingredients. Pour over pasta. Serve hot.

Serves 3-4

 We need to save every grain of food. There's a shortage of food worldwide.

VEGETABLES AND THAI NOODLES

½ pack flat rice noodles, boiled and drained

1 extra firm tofu, cubed

½ cup sesame oil

1 teaspoon cumin seeds

½ inch ginger, grated

½ cup Bragg's liquid amino acid

2 carrots, chopped

1 zucchini, chopped

1 celery, chopped

2 teaspoons tahini

½ cup lemon juice

½ bunch fresh mint

½ bunch fresh basil

salt to taste

black pepper to taste

In a pan, sauté tofu with sesame oil, cumin seeds, ginger and Bragg's on medium. Add carrots, zucchini and celery to the stir fry and cook. Season with salt and black pepper. When vegetables are slightly soft, add cooked noodles. Add tahini, lemon juice, fresh mint and basil. Serve hot.

Serves 3-4

 If we know what to eat, then we can protect ourselves from diseases.

PASTA WITH SUN-DRIED TOMATO SAUCE

2 tablespoons olive oil

1 zucchini, finely chopped

1 fresh tomato, finely chopped

2 tablespoons Italian herbs

1 tablespoon rosemary

salt to taste

black pepper to taste

½ cup pine nuts

½ cup sun-dried tomatoes

½ bunch fresh basil

salt to taste

black pepper to taste

½ cup olive oil

In a pan, heat olive oil on medium. Sauté zucchini and fresh tomato with Italian herbs, rosemary, salt and black pepper. For sauce, blend pine nuts, sun-dried tomatoes, basil, salt, pepper and olive oil in blender. Add the sauce to the vegetables and mix. Pour vegetables and sauce over whole wheat pasta. Garnish with fresh basil and serve hot.

Serves 3-4

 The type of food you take governs your mind. And again, your mind has a direct impact on your body. That is why you should eat food with a happy state of mind.

PESTO ZUCCHINI AND SQUASH PASTA

2 cups zucchini, shaved into long strips

2 cups yellow squash, shaved into long strips

3 tablespoons olive oil

salt to taste

1 cup pine nuts

½ cup fresh basil

½ cup lemon juice, freshly squeezed

1 teaspoon Bragg's liquid amino

1 cup tomatoes, finely chopped

1 cup red bell peppers, chopped

1 cup yellow bell peppers, chopped

1 cup broccoli, chopped

½ teaspoon black pepper

Shave zucchini and squash into lengthwise ribbons (like fettuccini pasta) using a vegetable peeler. Cook in two batches. In a pan, heat 1 tablespoon olive oil on medium-high. When hot, add first batch of zucchini and squash ribbons and salt to taste. Cook, tossing and stirring for 2 to 3 minutes, until softened and beginning to turn translucent. Transfer to a serving dish. Repeat with the remaining zucchini and squash.

For pesto, blend pine nuts, basil, lemon juice, Bragg's and a pinch of salt in blender until smooth. Add tomatoes and pulse until blended.

Heat 1 tablespoon olive oil in a pan, and sauté bell peppers and broccoli for several minutes. Add pesto from blender and zucchini and squash ribbons and toss. Cook on low heat for another 5 minutes. Season with black pepper to taste. Serve hot.

Serves 3-4

If we are very excited, we cannot swallow food with ease. Also, if we are restless, we end up eating more food. So, it is important to have food with awareness.

LENTILS

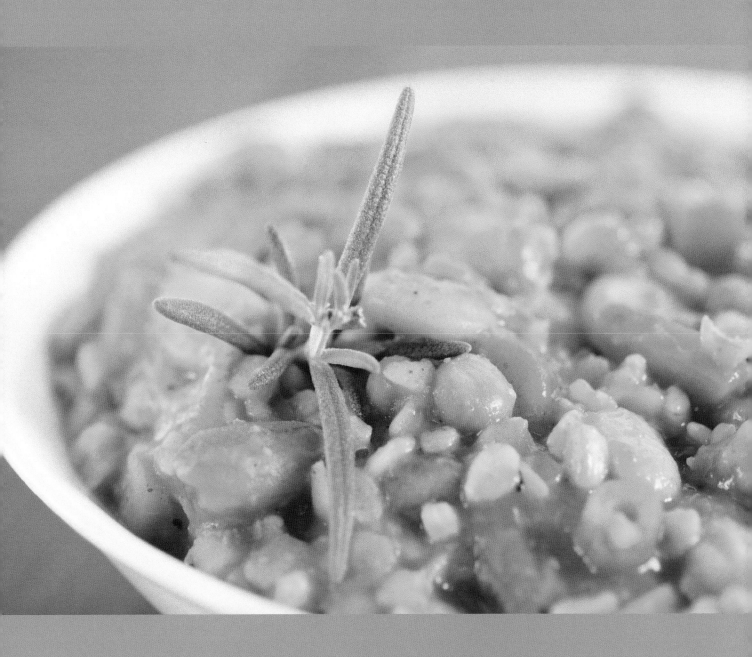

DAL (LENTILS)

1½ cups dal

6 cups water

2 tablespoons olive oil

¼ teaspoon mustard seeds

¼ teaspoon fenugreek seeds

5 whole cloves

¼ teaspoon cumin seeds

¼ teaspoon asafoetida

¼ teaspoon turmeric

1 green chili, chopped (optional)

1 teaspoon ginger, grated

1 teaspoon lemon juice

2 teaspoons jaggery (optional)

salt to taste

chopped coriander leaves for garnish

Wash, then soak dal for 2 hours. Cook dal in 6 cups water until very soft, roughly 30 minutes. In a separate pan, heat olive oil on medium and then add mustard, fenugreek and cloves. When mustard seeds pop, add cumin seeds and asafoetida. When heated, add turmeric, chili, ginger, and salt.

Pour dal into spice mixture and add water as needed to thin to desired consistency. Add lemon juice and jaggery. Cook thoroughly. Garnish with coriander. Serve with rice.

Serves 3-4

 Nature is such that it produces only those things which are good for that season. So the fruits, vegetables, and everything—nature has done it in such a way to suit us according to the time and season.

MASOOR DAL (SPLIT RED LENTILS)

1½ cups masoor dal

4 cups water

2 tablespoons olive oil

¼ teaspoon mustard seeds

1 teaspoon ground ginger

½ teaspoon coriander powder

1 teaspoon turmeric

6 whole cloves

1 stick cinnamon

salt to taste

Wash masoor dal and soak for one hour. In a pan, heat olive oil on medium and add mustard seeds. When mustard seeds pop, add ginger, coriander powder, turmeric, cloves and cinnamon. Add dal and water to pan. Cook until dal is very soft. Serve hot with rice.

Variation: Add ½ pound of chopped spinach near the end of cooking. Serve with rice.

Serves 3-4

 You know, usually people who overeat, they eat so fast. They stuff things so fast, but if you keep the food in your mouth, chew it longer, just feel the food in your mouth, you will see you will consume half of what you usually consume, yes?

BEANS, RICE, AND VEGETABLES

1 cup dried mung beans
¾ cup uncooked rice
2 cups mixed vegetables
1 cup green beans, chopped
2 tomatoes, chopped
2 tablespoons olive oil
¼ teaspoon mustard seeds
¼ teaspoon cumin seeds
¼ teaspoon fenugreek seeds
¼ inch ginger, grated
½ teaspoon red pepper flakes
¼ teaspoon turmeric
salt to taste
coriander for garnish

Wash and soak mung beans in water for one hour. In 2 cups of water, bring beans and rice to a boil, then simmer for seven minutes. When half done, add 2 cups mixed vegetables (whatever you like, e.g. carrots, potatoes, celery, zucchini, etc.) When almost cooked, add green beans and tomatoes.

In a separate pan, heat olive oil on medium and add mustard seeds. Once mustard seeds pop, add cumin seeds, fenugreek seeds, ginger, red pepper flakes, turmeric and salt. Add to the rice-bean-vegetable mixture and simmer for a few more minutes. Garnish with coriander. Serve hot with rice.

Serves 3-4

 A properly balanced diet has an impact on our emotions and thereby on our consciousness.

COCONUT QUINOA QUINOA

1 cup quinoa

½ cup masoor dal, washed and soaked

2 cups water

1 carrot

1 bell pepper

½ bunch baby spinach

1 tomato

½ inch ginger, grated

3 tablespoons olive oil or ghee

1 teaspoon cumin seeds

¼ teaspoon turmeric

½ cup coconut powder

salt to taste

black pepper to taste

chopped coriander leaves for garnish

Cook quinoa, masoor dal, vegetables and ginger with salt in a rice cooker or thick pot in 2 cups of water. Add extra water if necessary to make sure ingredients are soft and cooked through. In a pan, heat olive oil on medium and add cumin seeds. Roast cumin seeds until dark brown. Add turmeric and coconut powder. Add spice mixture to quinoa, dal and vegetable mixture. Add salt and black pepper to taste. Garnish with coriander.

Serves 3-4

 If you don't eat too much, then you are on the safe side. Too much food makes you feel dull. Meditation doesn't happen then.

CHICKPEA CURRY

3 tablespoons ghee or olive oil
1 teaspoon cumin seeds
½ inch ginger, grated
2 tomatoes, diced
1 teaspoon cumin powder
½ teaspoon garam masala
1 cup cooked chickpeas
½ cup lemon juice
coriander to garnish

In a pan, heat olive oil on medium, add cumin seeds and roast until brown. Then add ginger, diced tomatoes, cumin powder and garam masala. Add the cooked chickpeas to the spices, and salt to taste. Once soft, add lemon juice. Garnish with coriander. Serve hot with rice or bread.

Serves 3-4

 Observe nature, observe yourself - your own breath, your own body. And do it with the least amount of effort.

MUNG DAL AND SPINACH

1 cup mung dal

2 cups water

1 tablespoon olive oil or ghee

½ teaspoon mustard seeds

¼ teaspoon cumin seeds

¼ teaspoon asafoetida

¼ teaspoon turmeric powder

1 teaspoon coriander powder

¼ teaspoon cumin powder

1 teaspoon fresh ginger, grated

1 tablespoon lemon juice

salt to taste

1 cup spinach, chopped

½ teaspoon garam masala (optional)

Wash mung dal. Cook dal in 2 cups water until semi-cooked. In a pan, heat olive oil on medium and add mustard seeds. Once mustard seeds pop, add cumin seeds and asafoetida. Add turmeric powder, coriander powder, cumin powder and ginger. Add salt and lemon juice. Pour mung dal into the pan with the cooked spices. Mix spinach with the dal. Add garam masala, if preferred. Cook for about 10 minutes, until the dal is soft. Serve hot.

Serves 3-4

 Organic food is very good for [us]. It is a benefit to the farmers and is good for our health. Otherwise, they use so many chemicals to raise their crops, and then we complain of stomach ache and back ache.

DESSERTS

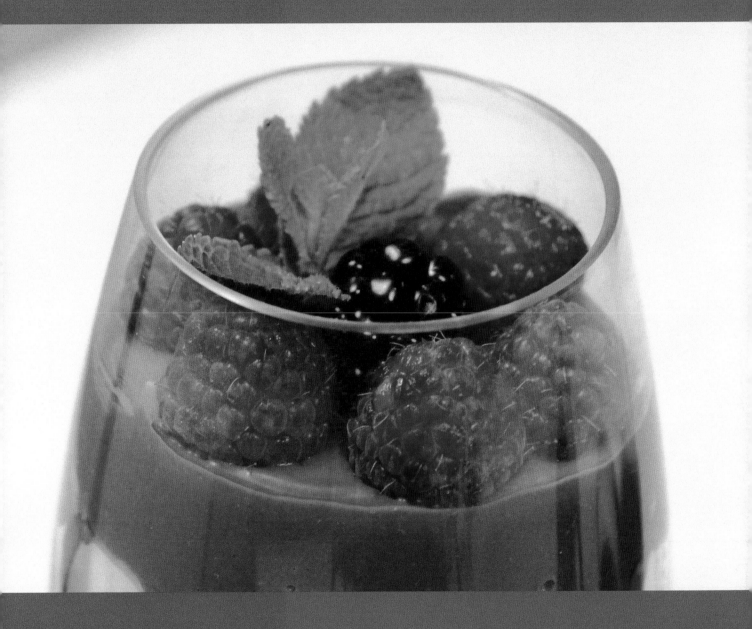

CHOCOLATE AVOCADO MOUSSE

2 large, ripe avocados, halved and pitted

½ cup cocoa powder

½ cup agave nectar

½ teaspoon vanilla extract

½ cup orange juice

fresh mixed berries and mint to garnish

Mix avocados with cocoa in a blender until smooth. Add orange juice, agave and vanilla extract and blend until mixture becomes one consistent color and texture. Pour into martini glasses and garnish with fresh berries and mint. Serve cool.

Serves 3-4

 Everything is alive in this universe in some way or another.

BLISS BALLS

½ cup dates, soaked
½ cup almonds
½ cup dry coconut powder

Mix dates and almonds in a blender and blend until smooth. Form mixture into small, round balls. Roll balls in coconut powder and serve.

Serves 3-4

 Thought is nothing but a quantum of energy and consciousness. Food absorbs thought. So, bless the food today for lunch. Don't think negative while eating. That is where the negative cycle begins.

LIVE APPLE PIE

½ cup dates, soaked
½ cup almonds, powdered
½ cup dry coconut powder
1 cup apples, chopped
½ cup raisins, soaked
½ teaspoon cinnamon
mixed berries to garnish

Blend soaked dates, powdered almonds and coconut powder together. Line a round pie dish with this "crust" around the walls and bottom. Blend apples, raisins and cinnamon together and fill the crust with the mixture. Garnish and decorate with coconut powder and fresh berries. Serve cool.

Serves 3-4

 Annadata Sukhi Bhava: 'Those who are providing me with this food, may they be happy.' Before eating food, you should say this once or twice.

APPLE CRUMB CAKE

6 macintosh apples, peeled and sliced

1 cup sugar

2 teaspoons cinnamon

1 stick butter, softened

½ cup brown sugar

1 cup wheat flour

¾ cup pecans, halved

Mix apples, sugar, and one teaspoon cinnamon together in a bowl. Blend butter, brown sugar and flour together separately. Add pecans and remaining teaspoon of cinnamon into flour mix. Butter a 9"x13" pan and pour apple mix into the pan. Sprinkle flour mix over the apples. Bake in pre-heated oven at 350 degrees for 50 to 60 minutes. Serve hot.

Serves 3-4

 If the farmers are happy, our body will be disease-free. So, bless the farmers, pray for the farmers.

CHOCOLATE COCONUT MACAROONS

3 cups unsweetened shredded coconut

2 tablespoons maple syrup

1½ cups cocoa powder

¼ teaspoon sea salt

1 teaspoon vanilla

1 tablespoon coconut butter

Mix all ingredients together and form into balls. Serve cool.

Serves 3-4

 Pay attention to your food.

Made in the USA
Charleston, SC
20 December 2012